AROMATHERAPY FOR CYNICS

Relax and Let Your Body Heal

Tamara J. Helms

TABLE OF CONTENTS

CHAPTER 1

WHAT IS AROMATHERAPY?

Sure, maybe you have heard of aromatherapy before and are, at least, marginally familiar with the term and the basics of what it means.

Aromatherapy has something to do with scents and smells treating illnesses and conditions, right? Now, that does sound a bit unbelievable! How can it possibly do that, simply through the smell of something?

Don't worry; you are not alone in your cynicism. Others have often questioned the viability of this treatment method. How is it supposed to work anyway? To better understand aromatherapy and how it works – if it does work at all – we need to understand better what aromatherapy truly is.

Aromatherapy is a generic term that refers to many different types of traditions that use plant matter and essential oils to create a more positive atmosphere in conjunction with benefiting someone's quality of life. Throughout the civilized Western world, all current treatments that use essential oils and plant matter are considered aromatherapy rather than "actual" medical treatments.

In general, aromatherapy is a form of therapy meant to help someone relax or reduce stress. Aromatherapy is practiced using essential oils and volatile plant oils to create psychological and physical sensations. It usually requires aromatic compounds produced through explosive plant materials, essential oils, or similar herbal products. It is used as a form of alternative medicine for positively affecting a person's health or mood.

All of these many uses have made aromatherapy a prevalent treatment method among alternative medicines. Many people who do not like the sometimes unpleasant side effects of prescribed medication, particularly for depression, stress, or other similar disorders, have opted to use aromatherapy to help reach the desired state of being. You might think of some of these people as oddballs for choosing to use aromatherapy instead of other synthetic medications. Still, it has proven to be effective in certain circumstances when used appropriately or with a physician's permission.

CHAPTER 2

HISTORY OF AROMATHERAPY

Aromatherapy has been used in one form or another for thousands of years. Throughout time, people have used essential oils and plant matter to heal illnesses and cure diseases. For this reason, it is hard to give a specific date or event timeline for the creation and development of aromatherapy. It has adjusted over time to meet the particular needs of each culture as the cultural needs have changed. It has also been modified as new plant matter and essential oils have been discovered and utilized.

Due to this ever-changing history, aromatherapy, in its current manifestation, evolved with distilled plant material to create essential oils. This particular form of distillation can be traced back to a 20th-century innovation.

As currently defined in the medical field, aromatherapy is a term that was first coined in 1920 by French chemist Renée Maurice Gattefosse.

This renowned French chemist Renee Maurice Gattefosse had dedicated his life to research and study regarding the healing properties of essential oils. This dedication was spurred by an incident that happened by chance in his laboratory one day. Gattefosse accidentally set his arm on fire and was racing around the inside of his lab, searching for some way to put the flames out. While searching for the nearest vat of liquid to thrust his arm into, French chemist Renée Maurice Gattefosse came across a large open container of lavender oil.

Quickly, the chemist put his arm into the lavender oil to extinguish the flames, and, to his surprise, he experienced almost instant pain relief.

Gattefosse also noticed through this life-changing experience that his burns healed remarkably quickly and left minimal scarring. The difference in the healing process between these burns that were slathered in lavender oil and the burns that the chemist had suffered regularly astonished him. One of the most significant breakthroughs that the French chemist Renée Maurice Gattefosse had discovered was that the lavender oil had shortened the overall healing process and healed with very little redness, inflammation, heat rashes, blisters, or scarring.

It was not until World War II that the French chemist Renée Maurice Gattefosse was continued through Jean Valnet. Jean Valnet had used essential oils and other distilled plant material to treat gangrene in wounded soldiers. While it was not necessarily a cure, there were many cases when Jean Valnet was capable of saving soldiers' lives using these essential oils – a beneficial discovery during wartime crises.

CHAPTER 3

DOES AROMATHERAPY WORK?

This is a persistent question among most people when they think about aromatherapy. Does Aromatherapy work, or is it all just a big sham? It is a common misperception that aromatherapy is new.

Aromatherapy has been in existence and recognized as such for at least 80 years. However, the essential nature of aromatherapy has existed for thousands of years.

To start with, do not get fooled by companies who will try to sell their pleasant smelling products as aromatherapy products. Some companies will excite unfounded claims to be aromatherapy to make more sales. In countries such as the United States, Aromatherapy is treated like other chemicals, and the FCC requires appropriate identification of all ingredients. Make sure that what you were looking at contains all-natural ingredients, not synthetic ones.

So what about significant illnesses? Can aromatherapy help with diseases or psychological problems? The truth of the matter is that aromatherapy cannot cure stress or cure a condition. Anyone who goes into the use of aromatherapy to fix something is going to be disappointed. This isn't how aromatherapy works.

However, aromatherapy is geared towards helping you cope with a physical condition and the symptoms of an illness, and improve your mood, temporarily ease stress, or help with other psychological diseases. This does not mean all of these symptoms or issues will go away. It simply means that aromatherapy can help make these symptoms and issues easier to deal with.

Aromatherapy is unable to cure cancer, AIDS, or other significant illnesses.

Instead, it can help calm the fear, reduce nausea, and enhance a person's overall mood. It should never be used as a primary treatment method for any major illness. It only acts as a complementary treatment that supports other treatments already ongoing.

It can offer the possibility of taking the place of prescription or over-the-counter chemical drugs in certain areas. For instance, it can substantially benefit in dealing with indigestion, inflammation, skincare, hygiene, wounds, and mental or emotional issues.

In addition, aromatherapy will not work the same way for each person who tries it. Your sensory memory is going to affect how or when therapy will work for you. Therefore, if you have a terrible experience with a particular sense, this will not have the correct impact on you as is desired.

Do some research on the company planning to buy your essential oils or other aromatherapy treatment ingredients. You want to make sure they are using all-natural ingredients and give you correct information on using the aromatherapy ingredients. For instance, be cautious of companies that tell you to use essential oils on your skin. You should only use essential oils on your skin if they are diluted. Many mislabeled products on the market and a tremendous amount of misinformation about aromatherapy may also make bogus claims about the so-called healing properties of aromatherapy oils.

CHAPTER 4

AROMATHERAPY AT HOME

Aromatherapy can be used as a form of treatment or prevention for some diseases and can be extremely useful for reducing stress levels. The essential oils released through aromatherapy have a significant influence on the aroma center of the brain, specifically in the limbic system. While no specific medical studies have proven aromatherapy to have positive effects on the body currently, many preliminary clinical studies show a synergy between the body's healing processes and aromatic oils. These aromatic oils are often released as gas or vapor during aromatherapy, as the fats are often burned.

Throughout the English-speaking world, aromatherapy is used on a day-to-day basis, even if you are not aware of it. Many people in Western civilizations may not necessarily recognize it as aromatherapy but are likely to see it in their day-to-day lives through perfumes, massage oils, and scented lotions. This is one reason why many practitioners emphasize their use of aromatherapy through massage oils and incense. It is only in America and other English-speaking countries that aromatherapy is regarded as such a complementary method.

Have you ever used perfume to get the desired scent? Have you ever used lotions that, for some reason, feel so soothing to you? Have you ever burned incense with names such as "Tranquility" found that the smell was quite soft and helped you to relax? Have you ever used bath soap or other bath lotion that was designed to help soothe and calm?

These are all aspects of aromatherapy in its complementary sense. These are methods through which people use scents, smells, and other natural elements to help create a soothing, warm, and welcoming environment.

In France, where it was initially discovered, aromatherapy is a part of their national mainstream medicine. Throughout France, there is an emphasis on using the many properties of essential oils such as antiseptic, antiviral, antifungal, and antibacterial properties. They may also find these properties to be in other distilled plant material and use these properties to control the spread of infections.

This is quite different from the methods familiar to many English-speaking countries. In France and its neighboring countries, it is not uncommon for a patient to be prescribed essential oils that a physician administers.

Can you imagine what that would be like in the United States? Imagine if you were going to a physician who prescribed you an aromatherapy treatment for your stress, rather than synthetic medication. This would indeed be different from what we are accustomed to in Western civilizations. Yet, so many other countries use aromatherapy treatments to prevent illnesses and treat existing diseases or conditions.

Although there have been many breakthroughs throughout the aromatherapy medicine field, present-day aromatherapy is a form of a valid science branch that has not been validated in the United States, Russia, Germany, or Japan. It is prevalent for physicians in these countries to neglect to recognize the usefulness of aromatherapy treatments. Yet, other countries worldwide are still using aromatherapy to treat illnesses and diseases and prevent further infection of conditions or diseases. Despite the apparent usefulness of aromatherapy and reducing stress levels, most physicians in Western civilizations do not like to use aromatherapy in treating stress.

CHAPTER 5

WHAT EFFECTS DOES AROMATHERAPY
HAVE ON THE LIMBIC SYSTEM?

Perhaps the use of aromatherapy may not be so apparent to you either. It is helpful to understand how aromatherapy works to know how it can help. The primary effects of aromatherapy are on the limbic system. The medical community has described the limbic system as a set of brain structures that support various functions. The functions that the limbic system of the brain maintains include both the motion and memory brain functions. This system of the brain operates in tandem with the endocrine system and the automatic nervous system. Through the endocrine system, the limbic system can influence the amount of pleasure that is felt. The same part of the brain plays a role in sexual arousal and other high-endorphin moments.

Because of the significant role that a scent can play in bringing specific memories or emotions, aromatherapy can be a helpful tool to utilize or apply therapy to the brain's limbic system.

There are various aromatherapy scents and related feelings to these scents; the smells are designed to remind the person taking them of a happy time or place that the person has had at some point within their life. That limbic system response is why many aromatherapy products have some success using smells that are season-oriented. Often, the cinnamon candle can remind someone of Christmas or give him or her all of the Christmas season feelings.

Have you ever wondered why a certain sense of smell will remind you of places, people, or things? Have you ever noticed that some smells will make you feel warm and comfortable, remind you of places where you were happy, and other scents can have the opposite effect?

This is very similar to how aromatherapy works. The scents and smells will evoke specific responses within your body that will produce the desired effect.

CHAPTER 6

ESSENTIAL OILS

How to determine what essential oils are best.

Many essential oils can be used in aromatherapy. There are at least 90 different essential oils and absolutes and at least 15 carrier oils commonly used in aromatherapy. With so many other oils to choose from, it is no wonder that most people have difficulty understanding what oils may be best for their specific desired effect. It is essential to study the different oil types to determine which one will be the best one to use, should you decide to use aromatherapy.

Undiluted essential oils and similar products suitable for aromatherapy can usually be distinguished from other similar products since, in most cases, the pure oils are of a therapeutic grade. This, of course, is only an excellent standard to go on if you live in a country that regulates the industry. In the United States, the content of oil components is standardized to the use of FCC labeling. FCC labeling refers to the food chemical codex. A criterion established by the FCC determines the specified amounts of a specific aroma, and creating chemicals must naturally occur in the oil.

This type of regulation is used to help regulate the industry so that aromatherapy retains at least some sense of standards. Not only does the FCC help to regulate aromatherapy, but it also helps determine what types of oils and essential plant material are best suited for specific therapies. In addition, this regulation determines how much clear oil should be used for a particular purpose, eliminating the worry of using too much of a specific oil. However, no law prevents a manufacturer from adding a synthetic chemical to meet any criteria established by the FCC in any particular oil.

However, the best method for determining if an essential oil will be of much use is simply an educated nose. Many people specifically skilled in aromatherapy can often determine if a scent is synthetic or natural. This skill is believed anyone can obtain as long as he or she is willing to put in the time and effort. You must try to avoid adulterated oils and materials for your aromatherapy whenever possible.

No matter what therapy, sense, or smell you end up choosing, you must remain close to your natural preference. In many cases, if you like how an oil smells or makes you feel, more than likely, you will enjoy using it. If you do not want the smell and enjoying using it as a form of therapy, it will do you no good, regardless of what that specific oil or scent is supposed to do or how it 10

should benefit you. If you are not enjoying the smell of one particular essential oil, this is your body's way of telling you to keep looking.

How to test an essential oil

When you sample various types of essential oils for your aromatherapy, you must test them properly. To sample an oil, open the bottle approximately 3 to 4 inches directly below your nose. Slowly sway the bottle from right to left as you gently inhale. You mustn't inhale too deeply or use the bottle as an inhaler. Breathing the aroma more deeply will not increase potency and could be dangerous as specific oils can have an overpowering smell.

It would help determine what oils feel most natural to you and what oils bring about specific feelings within you through this sampling. As I mentioned before, people often associate the smell of cinnamon with the holiday season, and the same can be said for the scent of pine trees and campfires. While there is undoubtedly no essential oil for campfires, there is for pine trees and just about any other season or experience, you would like to conjure up.

What are essential oils?

Essential oil is usually a liquid that has been derived from a plant and distilled. This distilling process usually involves water from a stream or slow-moving river combined with the leaves, flowers, stems, bark, and other parts of the plant used to make this particular oil. Essential oils do not feel oily at all, contrary to the use of the word. Most essential oils are transparent or are a transparent orange or amber color. Essential oils are believed to contain the true essence of the plant or tree from which they were obtained. Due to the high concentration that the vital oils maintain, they are often sold in tiny bottles that can last a long time.

Essential oils, while they do represent scents, are not the same or even similar to fragrances or perfumes. Essential oils are always derived from natural plants. In contrast, the vast majority of perfume or fragrance oils are artificially created or, at the very least, contain artificial substances and often offer little or no therapeutic value. Since the use of the word aromatherapy is not yet regulated by the United States government, many companies will provide fragrance oils as aromatherapy therapeutic oils even though they are not the same.

This is an unfortunate situation as many times; these fragrant oils have little or no natural ingredients. It is essential to understand that if an aromatherapy product contains any synthetic or perfume oil, it is not an actual aromatherapy product, simply someone trying to sell a lesser product as a greater one.

The aroma and chemical composition of therapeutic essential oils is the key. This makes aroma and chemical composition can provide valuable physical therapeutic benefits and psychological stress relief. The majority of people who practice therapeutic oils do so through methods, including diluting oil to the skin and through inhalation.

The major essential oils

There are many different types of essential oils, and all of them have specific properties. You may not even realize it, but many of these oils are used in their other forms while cooking! For example, some of the following essential oils are ones you would find in everyday household cooking in a different format (such as leaves or ground powder):

Basil

Basil is often used in cooking for various purposes because of its unique flavor. Its aromatic properties are sweet, herbaceous, and licorice-like. While basil is most often used in cooking, it can help treat bronchitis, colds, coughs, exhaustion, flatulence, flu, gout, insect bites, insect repellent, muscle aches, rheumatism, and sinusitis. However, it is suggested that basil only be used sparingly and with caution. Too much basil may be carcinogenic because it contains methyl chavicol. It is recommended that you do not use basil if you have liver problems, and you should not use basil during pregnancy.

Ginger

Ginger, also often used in cooking, is another aromatherapy essential oil. It has a warm, spicy, earthy, and woodsy smell. Ginger is best used to treat aching muscles, arthritis, nausea, and poor circulation.

However, you should not use this if you will be exposed to direct sunlight for an extended period to create sun poisoning.

Lemon

Lemon is a ubiquitous fruit that most people are familiar with. Its aroma is very similar to the scent of lemon rinds except more affluent and more concentrated. It can be used to treat athlete's foot, chilblains, colds, corns, dull skin, flu, oily skin, spots, varicose veins, and warts.

Like Ginger, it is suggested that lemon not be used if you will be exposed to direct sunlight for an extended period.

Parsley

Parsley is also often used in cooking. It has a very woodsy aroma that can be pretty appealing. It is often used to treat amenorrhea, arthritis, cellulite, cystitis, frigidity, griping pains, indigestion, rheumatism, and toxic build-up. However, this particular essential oil can sometimes be 12

dangerous. It tends to be harmful to the liver and can induce abortions. It should be used in each with extreme caution, particularly around pregnant women.

Peppermint

Peppermint is a pervasive smell that you are probably very familiar with. It is minty and is very reminiscent of spearmint, only more concentrated and fragrant. This scent will often remind people of the Christmas holiday. It is an excellent treatment for asthma, colic, exhaustion, fever, flatulence, headache, nausea, scabies, sinusitis, and vertigo. It can be somewhat toxic to the nerves and should be avoided in someone afflicted with epilepsy or fever. Peppermint may be taken orally but only under the guidance of a qualified aromatherapy practitioner.

Thyme

Thyme is frequently used in cooking. It has a fresh but medicinal type smell. Thyme is often used to treat arthritis, colds, cuts, dermatitis, flu, insect bites, laryngitis, lice, muscle aches, oily skin, poor circulation, scabies, and sore throats.

People with hypertension should not use thyme. It can also cause dermal irritation or can be a solid mucous membrane irritant.

Rose

Exciting is the use of Rose in Aromatherapy. All of us are accustomed to roses being used as a gift. However, roses are also used for aromatherapy. They have a floral and sweet sense. Rose is often used to treat depression, eczema, frigidity, mature skin, menopause, and stress in its essential oil form. When you think of giving roses to someone you care about, remember that just the scent of roses can help to alleviate depression and anxiety. No wonder women like them so much.

Nutmeg

Most everyone is very familiar with nutmeg. It has a beautiful smell that is rich, spicy, sweet, and woodsy. The essential oil is very similar to that of the cooking spice, only more affluent and more fragrant. It is commonly used to treat arthritis, constipation, fatigue, muscle aches, nausea, neuralgia, poor circulation, rheumatism, and slow digestion.

Marjoram

Marjoram is also a cooking spice, the only one not used as frequently as others mentioned here. In its aromatherapy version, its sweet and woodsy smell can be very appealing. It can deal with a vast number of potential problems while still smelling nice.

It is used to treat aching muscles, amenorrhea, bronchitis, chilblains, 13 colic, coughing, excessive sex drive, flatulence, hypertension, muscle cramps, neuralgia, rheumatism, sprains, strains, stress, and ticks.

However, pregnant women should avoid using it, although there are no other precautions necessary.

Lavender

Earlier, in the history of aromatherapy, it was mentioned that the French chemist Gattefosse discovered aromatherapy through an accidental dosage of Lavender oil. What does lavender treat?

Its fresh, sweet, floral, and slightly fruity scent is much enjoyed. Its possible uses are many and include acne, allergies, anxiety, asthma, athlete's foot, bruises, burns, chickenpox, colic, cuts, cystitis, depression, dermatitis, dysmenorrheal, earache, flatulence, headache, hypertension, insect bites, insect repellant, itching, labor pains, migraine, oily skin, rheumatism, scabies, scars, sores, sprains, strains, stress, stretch marks, vertigo, and whooping cough. Even with all its many treatments, there is no need for special precautions with this essential oil.

Essential Oil Safety

Like all treatments, medications, and therapies, you must exercise safety and caution when using essential oils.

Remember that these are highly concentrated liquids, which can be harmful if they are not used as prescribed or appropriately. However, do not let that scare you. Just as long as you exercise caution and stay informed, you should do just fine with aromatherapy.

While some safety guidelines should be followed, they can sometimes be broken under the guidance of a qualified and trained aromatherapy practitioner in the case of certain oils. When in doubt, always consult your physician or a skilled and experienced aromatherapy practitioner.

An important guideline to remember is an essential oil should never be used undiluted on the skin. While there may be exceptions to this precaution, you should never make that judgment on your own without careful consultation with authority on the subject. Using the oil on the skin can cause skin irritation, rashes, severe sensitivity, and toxicity. Lavender and tea tree can be used on the skin but should only be done so on infrequent occasions so that you do not incur the possibility of sensitivity.

Keep in mind that some oils may produce sensitivity or allergic reactions in some individuals. Like with almost all other things, some people are bound to be allergic to essential oils used in aromatherapy.

To safeguard yourself and others against a potential allergic 14 reaction, always apply a minimal amount of diluted essential oil (never undiluted) onto a small skin patch. It can be helpful to do this on the inside of an elbow and then apply Band-Aid. Allow the oil to sit for at least 24 hours to see any form of reaction. It does not matter if you think you will not be allergic to any essential oil; you should always check first.

Some essential oils will also be problematic for people during pregnancy or those with asthma, epilepsy, or other severe health conditions. Keep this in mind and look for precautions on that essential oil before using it with a person who has a potential health issue to prevent complications.

Never take essential oils orally unless under specific directions from a physician or qualified aromatherapy practitioner. Most oils cannot be taken orally, but a rare few can in typical regulated doses. A physician or qualified aromatherapy practitioner should only prescribe these.

Unlike most things in life, essential oils are always falling under the rule of less is more. Use only a tiny amount of essential oil, just enough to get the job done. Essential oils are highly concentrated, and it is straightforward to use too much.

Not everything that is an essential oil should be used for aromatherapy. Certain essential oils such as wormwood, pennyroyal, onion, camphor, horseradish, wintergreen, rue, bitter almond, and sassafras should only be used under the direction of or by a qualified aromatherapy practitioner if it is used at all

Keep in mind that essential oils are flammable! Always keep essential oils away from fire hazards, and you should use extreme caution when the oils are near flames.

It should go without saying that you should never let children use essential oils without the presence of an adult who is versed in information about aromatherapy. However, we may neglect to remember to take this precaution by preventing children from getting into your essential oils store. Keep them somewhere safe and out of a child's reach.

CHAPTER 7

SAFETY FOR USERS

Are Aromatherapy Ingredients ok to use on pets?

Just as aromatherapy can be good for humans, it can also help our pets and provide them with the needed healing (both emotional and therapeutic) effects of aromatherapy. However, it is essential to remember that animals are much different from humans.

It is best to consult a qualified aromatherapy practitioner familiar with and comfortable working with animals. A recommended book on this topic is "Holistic Aromatherapy for Animals" by Kristen Leigh Bell, written in 2002. This book is the only primary resource on how aromatherapy affects animals.

Is Aromatherapy Safe for Children?

If you intend to use aromatherapy with your children, keep in mind that most recipes and guidelines currently available with aromatherapy are intended for normal, healthy, average-sized adults under the supervision of a medical professional. Any recipes designed to be used with children should have a significantly lower dosage than the standard formula would call for. Certain oils should not be used with children at all. It is better to be careful in this instance, and you should always use precaution and care when using aromatherapy treatments with children.

Some oils usually ok with children in small doses include neroli, rose, sweet orange, tea tree, lavender, and roman chamomile.

Children need to have specific considerations for age, size, weight, and needs, so it is best to consult a qualified person in these matters.

Should Pregnant Women use aromatherapy?

This is a highly debated subject. Many people do not feel aromatherapy should be used with pregnant women as the possible side effects are unknown in some cases, and there is little desire to

"test" this out to see if fetuses will be negatively affected by aromatherapy. Some people advise that certain oils are ok to use, and, indeed, a pregnant woman should never use some oils.

Some oils can cause spontaneous abortions or uterine contractions.

Other oils cause problems because they are bad for diabetics – and some pregnant women will develop diabetes during pregnancy. It is unclear, however, whether these oils were used appropriately and adequately when the incidences occurred.

Much of this research has been conducted on animals, as it is unsafe to do this type of testing on human beings. However, researchers have managed to identify some oils that are known to cause complications during pregnancy. These include:

Benzoin

Lemon

Sandalwood

Bergamot

Neroli

Spearmint

Grapefruit

Orange

Tea Tree

Lavender

Patchouli

Vetiver

Avoid these oils if you are pregnant or at risk of becoming pregnant. It is much better to find alternatives and be safe rather than sorry later down the road.

However, some aromatherapy oils are suitable for pregnant women. For instance, jasmine, clary sage, and rose tend to be very beneficial during the actual delivery even though they are not recommended for use during the actual pregnancy. It is best to have a qualified aromatherapist create a blend just for you to use during your delivery to help ease the pain, stress, and difficulties.

CHAPTER 8

CARRIER OILS

What are Carrier Oils?

Carrier oils are another part of aromatherapy treatment. While they are generally considered as base oils or vegetable oils, they have a more generalized purpose. Carrier oils are used to dilute essential oils, CO_2's, and absolutes before applying them onto your skin. This allows you to cut critical oil, combine it with a base oil or carrier oil, and be considered weak. This will make it safe for you to put it on your skin.

Different carrier oils offer other properties and can have therapeutic benefits of their own or increase the therapeutic benefit of the essential oil you are using. They are usually made from cold-pressed vegetable oils that are made from the fatty portions of certain plants. They do not evaporate or add their aroma to the essential oils. Interestingly, carrier oils can go wrong. While essential oils can last almost indefinitely, common carrier oils will expire. You want your carrier oils to be natural or to have natural vitamin E. added as a preservative.

Examples of carrier oils and their uses?

There are many different types of carrier oils. These are some of the more commonly used carrier oils.

Olive oil

Olive oil is often used in cooking. Its natural aroma is very close to that of the oil used in cooking, which means that it smells like olives. Its texture is heavy and somewhat oily, and it has a light to medium green color. It is essential to use a minimal amount or an appropriate amount in dilution to overpower the blend.

Peanut oil

Peanut oil has a high light aroma with a faintly nutty quality. Its texture is thick and leaves a very oily film on the skin, and its color is almost transparent. Use caution with peanut oil as it should not be used on anyone who has an allergy to peanuts. It is often a perfect choice to use with massage oils or in a massage blend because of its oily texture and help with arthritis.

Sweet Almond oil

Sweet almond oil has a light and slightly sweet, and nutty aroma. It is somewhat oily and will leave an oily feeling on the skin, but it absorbs quickly. It is virtually transparent but with a tinge of yellow. Sweet almond oil is an all-purpose carrier oil that can be used with almost any 19 essential oil and is moderately priced, making it an excellent choice for most essential oils.

Cocoa Butter Oil

Cocoa butter oil has a rich and sweet aroma that smells like chocolate. This type of butter remains solid and hard at room temperature and breaks into pieces. However, it is a good oil for heating and easing in lukewarm or warm weather. Its coloring is faintly tan. Cocoa butter oil should be blended with other materials or oils to be usable. It is an excellent oil to mix in for lotions and creams.

Hazelnut Oil

Hazelnut oil has a light, nutty, and somewhat sweet aroma. It is thin and leaves a very slightly oily feel. It is excellent to use for people who have oily skin as it does not go nearly as oily a residue as other carrier oils can. Not leaving an oily residue means the people using it will not have to suffer from acne breakouts quite often, which affects a large amount of the population in the United States and worldwide due to oil make-up's and oil residue leaving products.

Pecan Oil

Pecan oil has a faintly fatty and nutty aroma and has a medium thickness, leaving only a slight oily film on the skin. Its coloring is nearly precise, but it is said to go rancid fairly quickly. It needs to be stored in a dark-colored bottle in a dark area to protect it from exposure to sunlight, which will cause it to go wrong.

There is a wide variety of other carrier oils that you can use, and each one has its particular purpose, aroma, texture, and color. This list is not exhaustive but does give you a good understanding of potential oils that you can use to dilute your essential oils.

CHAPTER 9

OTHER MATERIALS

Absolutes?

Absolutes are very similar to essential oils. They are highly aromatic liquids, which have been extracted from plant material. However, the difference between essential oils and absolutes is that absolutes are extracted using a very complex method. It does require the use of chemical solvents that will later be removed during the final stages of production.

Absolutes tend to be more highly concentrated than their counterparts the essential oils are. This is why it is necessary to use crucial 20 healing oils in your treatment if you are using aromatherapy as a medical treatment or as a method to relax.

The major disadvantage of using absolutes or creating absolutes is those trace elements remain of the chemical solvent in the final product. This cannot be helped, as there is no way to ascertain that all chemical solvents have been removed from the absolute before reaching the final project stages. This is why many people use absolutes only sparingly because they are not 100% natural since they had to be extracted using chemical solvents.

One other significant difference between essential oils and absolutes is that the essential oils must be taken internally, except by educated, trained, and experienced enough. However, this is even more severe in the case of absolutes, which should never be taken internally, no matter who you are. The trace chemical material in the absolutes makes this a certainty.

Hydrosols?

Hydrosols are another ingredient that can be used in aromatherapy treatments. Hydrosols are the waters that remain after extracting essential oil from plant material. This is often referred to as floral water or distillate water. When extracting essential oil from plant material, the water itself will become infused with the beautiful aroma and some of the therapeutic properties of the oil itself. However, hydrosols are byproducts of the distillation process.

Resins?

You may be familiar with the term of resins already. Resin is a substance that occurs naturally when a tree is damaged. If the bark is pierced, trees will produce a thick, solid, sticky substance called resin. This resin is used for many different things, such as making figurines or other collectible items.

Resins produced naturally from trees do provide therapeutic benefits.

However, it can be challenging to work with these resins because of their thick and sticky nature. Liquid forms of resins can be found that have been extracted using a solvent or alcohol extraction technique.

CO2s?

CO2s are oils that have been extracted through a different method.

This method includes the use of carbon dioxide. Carbon dioxide is pressurized until it becomes a liquid. It is then capable of being used as a solvent on natural plant material, and the content of the plant that would have made essential oil dissolves into the liquid CO_2. Later on, 21 the concoction is drawn back up to its natural state, and the CO_2 particles evaporate into a gaseous state, leaving the resulting oil.

Typically, CO_2s are also interpreted as essential oils because there is no trace of any harmful solvent or chemical product left in the end product. This method does not diminish the potency of the oil either. CO_2s are generally thicker and more closely resemble the natural aroma of the original plant material. They are often sought out as a better product.

Infused Oils?

Another type of oil that is commonly used in aromatherapy is called infused oil. Infused oil uses a different method to extract the oils from plant material. In this method of extraction, carrier oil is permeated with one or more herbs.

This type of oil has carrier oil properties, but it also contains therapeutic properties of both the oil and the herbs infused into the oil.

While many plants contain healing or therapeutic properties, not all of these plants can be turned into essential oils. This is because they do not have enough oil material to extract for essential oil. However, this is why you would infuse that particular plant or herb with a carrier oil to making infused oil.

Infused oils are generally very oily, depending on what the base oil was. They are diluted as they have been combined with the carrier oil, and they can go bad over time. You can even make infused oil at home with a crock top at a shallow heat setting. It is easy to overheat the oil, so you have to be extremely careful when creating your own infused oil.

CHAPTER 10

USING AROMATHERAPY TO PROMOTE EMOTIONAL WELL-BEING

Introduction

Aromatherapy, particularly in essential oils, can be extremely useful in promoting solid emotional well-being. It can help promote positive emotional states of being and assist in dealing with grief, anger, or frustration. People who experience stress daily should consider using essential oils daily to help promote a less stressful environment to calm their nerves.

Aromatherapy works so well in this particular situation because essential oils are comprised of chemicals that occur naturally in plant material. That can be introduced in synergy with each other.

Their molecules are easily inhaled, allowing them to be fast-acting and be absorbed into the body quickly.

The molecules released through aromatherapy will stimulate and affect portions of the brain. The triggers that it provides to the brain can produce specific emotions or mask other types of emotions. Naturally, not all essential oils will affect everyone in the same manner. Other memories associated with particular kinds of aromas may affect how the scent will impact their emotional state.

For instance, if you have a robust emotional response to a specific type of oil or scent, this will affect its ability to influence your emotional well-being positively. If cinnamon, usually a warm and comforting scent, has become associated with the death of a family member, you are less likely to be positively influenced by cinnamon.

What essential oils influence emotional well-being?

It is believed by those who practice aromatherapy that it can significantly influence and improve a person's emotional well-being. We, as human beings, experience a wide variety of emotional states, and we need to address these emotional states to continue functioning in society. It is hard to deal with other people when stricken with grief – even more, when stricken with anger.

Therefore, some people turn to aromatherapy as a method to deal with these intense emotions. Different oils have properties that deal with other emotional states.

The list below covers most human emotions that we wish either to suppress or to enhance.

Anger

Grief

Bergamot, Jasmine, Neroli,

Cypress, Frankincense,

Orange, Patchouli, Petitgrain,

Helichrysum, Neroli, Rose,

Roman Chamomile, Rose,

Sandalwood, Vetiver

Vetiver, Ylang Ylang

Happiness and Peace

Anxiety

Bergamot, Frankincense,

Bergamot, Cedarwood, Clary

Geranium, Grapefruit, Lemon,

Sage, Frankincense, Geranium,

Neroli, Orange, Rose,

Lavender, Mandarin, Neroli,

Sandalwood, Ylang Ylang

Patchouli, Roman Chamomile,

Insecurity

Rose, Sandalwood, Vetiver

Bergamot, Cedarwood,

Confidence

Frankincense, jasmine,

Bay Laurel, Bergamot, Cypress,

Sandalwood, Vetiver

Grapefruit, Jasmine, Orange,

Irritability

Rosemary

Lavender, Mandarin, Neroli,

Depression

Roman Chamomile, Sandalwood

Bergamot, Clary Sage,

Loneliness

Frankincense, Geranium,

Grapefruit, Helichrysum,

Bergamot, Clary Sage,

Jasmine, Lavender, Lemon,

Frankincense, Helichrysum,

Mandarin, Neroli, Orange,

Roman Chamomile, Rose

Roman Chamomile, Rose,

Memory and Concentration

Sandalwood, Ylang Ylang

Basil, Black Pepper, Cypress,

Fatigue, Exhaustion and

Hyssop, Lemon, Peppermint,

Burnout

Rosemary

Basil, Bergamot, Black Pepper,

Panic and Panic Attacks

Clary Sage, Cypress,

Frankincense, Helichrysum,

Frankincense, Ginger,

Lavender, Neroli, Rose

Grapefruit, Helichrysum,

Jasmine, Lemon, Patchouli,

Stress

Peppermint, Rosemary,

Benzoin, Bergamot, Clary Sage,

Sandalwood, Vetiver

Frankincense, Geranium,

Grapefruit, Jasmine, Lavender,

Fear

Mandarin, Neroli, Patchouli,

Bergamot, Cedarwood, Clary

Roman Chamomile, Rose,

Sage, Frankincense, Grapefruit,

Sandalwood, Vetiver, Ylang

Jasmine, Lemon, Neroli,

Ylang

Orange, Roman Chamomile

Sandalwood, Vetiver

How does aromatherapy help depression?

In most cases, depression is caused by hormonal or chemical imbalances or through situational triggers. A "situational" trigger includes the death of a loved one, physical or verbal abuse, financial hardships, moving, loneliness, retirement, unemployment, divorce, or pressure in life. For most people, depression is short-lived and passes quickly, but other instances of depression may linger much longer.

If you believe that you have depression, it is always best to consult a qualified physician to address these issues. He or she will probably recommend therapy to you, and you may need to start taking medications. It is best to deal with depression under a physician's supervision.

If you decide to use aromatherapy to help with your depression, remember that it is only complementary. Aromatherapy can be beneficial in improving your overall mood and outlook on life. Still, it is no substitute for medical treatments to address your depression issues, mainly when hormonal or chemical imbalances cause them.

However, you can use aromatherapy to enhance your sense of well-being. Try using a diffuser (such as a reed diffuser where the oils climb a reed and diffuse into the air) during the day, an air freshener or room spray with aromatherapy ingredients, a massage with aromatherapy lotions (even a self-massage using aromatherapy oils can be so refreshing), skin, and hair aromatherapy products. Various instances where your senses are exposed to the oils' therapeutic properties will help make your day easier and help relieve your stress and anxiety. You can also use bath oils and bath salts.

CHAPTER 11

CAN AROMATHERAPY HELP
WITH WEIGHT LOSS?

Aromatherapy has been a highly debatable topic when it comes to weight loss. With everyone seeking a quick fix solution for obesity, every avenue has been turned to as a possible method for weight loss.

Like with all aspects of aromatherapy, there has been some degree of success, according to variables.

Like all weight loss programs, you need to consult a medical doctor or practitioner before setting up any weight loss plan for yourself. It is best to work with someone knowledgeable in this field to ensure that a project will be set up that addresses your specific needs.

Naturally, the use of essential oils will not make you shed pounds miraculously. Nothing will make you shed pounds miraculously, no matter what it says. However, aromatherapy can help to reduce your need to eat by decreasing your hunger and reducing your desire to eat more food. It can also help provide more incredible energy when working out and reduce your tiredness to feel more inclined to get up and exercise.

Any weight loss program requires eating the right food and plenty of exercises; keep this in mind when you are setting up your workout plan, as it is essential to stay on a schedule when trying to lose weight. All other items added to your diet plan are simply complementary to help you achieve your overall goal.

CHAPTER 12

WHAT IS ESSENTIAL OIL BLENDING?

Introduction

One unique and exciting thing about essential oils is that they can be blended to evoke specific responses in those exposed to the oils. You can easily create your essential oil blend to create a beautiful aromatic blend for your enjoyment and room fragrance. Essential oils can also be blended for therapeutic reasons to help ease muscles, reduce stress, or increase happiness. There are two significant reasons for blending critical oils: Aromatic and Therapeutic.

In aromatic blends, the focus is on the aroma of the final product.

While some aromatic blends will create therapeutic effects, the focus is to create a specific scent or smell for a particular purpose. Only natural ingredients should be used, such as absolutes, grain alcohol, carrier oils, essential oils, water, or herbs.

Most people work to produce a type of aroma such as a woodsy, earthy, spicy, citrus, floral, medicinal, minty, spicy, or Oriental aroma.

Be careful to analyze the aromatic properties of the essential oils you are using to ensure that they will not contradict each other too much. This will also be an excellent way to determine which essential oils are spicy, minty, or woodsy.

However, you do not need to stay within the same type of qualification of aroma to produce an excellent set. For instance, spicy and Oriental oils tend to go very well with floral, Orientals, or citrus oils as long as they are not overpowering. Floral oils tend to blend very well with spicy, citrus, and woodsy oils; keep this in mind when you are making an oil combination, as these oils could help you relax more and provide you with better treatment. Many different combinations can be used. To figure out which one of these works best for you, it is best to check many different aromatherapy combinations before deciding which one would work best.

In therapeutic blends, the focus is on the therapeutic effect of the mix. These blends are designed to help a physical condition or emotional state. You want to blend oils with the desired medicinal uses (such as treating asthma). You can combine multiple essential oils that have recommended pieces for treating asthma. This is not to be used as your regular treatment for asthma; when having an asthma attack, it would be essential to use your inhaler as the first piece of therapy, along then with aromatherapy 27 which will help calm down the asthma attack and future asthma attacks.

You can also blend essential oils with different properties to treat something like a combination of asthma, hypertension, arthritis, and insomnia. Just be careful not to also combine it with any essential oil that will hurt your health, and be very careful if you are pregnant or allergic to peanuts.

Consider as well that some essential oils are energizing oils while other oils will cause sleepiness. If you intend to use your oil before starting your day, do not use oils that are likely to make you fall asleep. This also works in reverse, so make sure that you are not using energizing oils right before you go to sleep, as this can cause you to stay up most of the night and leave you not rested enough to return to work as an actor and production person while you are visiting work the following day.

Blending oils to treat various illnesses or medical conditions is an excellent way to address your requirements precisely. Just be careful as you make your blends and try not to use too much of an overpowering type of oil which will cause it to be difficult for you to feel the effects of the other oils in the mix.

How do you blend?

There are no generally accepted rules to blending essential oils to produce a particular aroma or therapeutic combination.

However, there are some essential tips that you might want to consider when you are working on blending your oils. It is best to start using a small number of drops of each type of oil because a smaller amount will help you prevent wasting any oil unnecessarily. It also will help you to determine if more is less or less is more and figure out which one would be right for you.

You should first start your blend with just essential oils, absolutes, or CO_2s. You can then dilute it with other carrier oils or alcohol if you need to, which will help you prevent wasting any of your carrier oils or alcohol. Ensure that you keep a detailed list of each oil you are using and the number of drops used for that oil. It is too easy to get carried away and forget to take down these careful notes, but you will need these notes to duplicate your work later on, or if you want it and change it and make the recipe better.

Label your blends very carefully to know exactly what they are, what they are for, and what they have in them. You may also 28 consider putting some other kind of identification to your blend and keeping that identification with the recipe in some type of notebook.

Make sure that you are very careful about using oils that have an overpowering aroma. Certain aromas will be stronger than others and may overpower the rest if not used in the appropriate combination. You may want to consider experimenting with the oils before combining them with others so that you are aware of how strong the scent is and how strong its effect might be.

Even if you do not like your blend right away, it is not a good idea to destroy it. You should hang onto the mix for a little while and revisit it at a later date. Sometimes, the ingredients in your blend will need time to settle to invoke the right aroma. Besides, you may get used to it! You might also have been exposed to too many intense aromas before your 'questionable' product was complete, thereby making it difficult to get a good sense of the natural smell.

CHAPTER 13

DIFFUSERS?

A diffuser is a 'tool' that you can use as a method of helping diffuse the molecules of essential oil into the air. The diffuser enables you to best use the aromatherapy treatment's effects as you breathe in your ordinary air.

Tissues

One of the simplest methods of diffusion is through tissue or handkerchief. The tissue has several tiny drops of oil placed onto it, but this tissue will carry the molecules wherever you take the tissue.

It is incredibly portable and can be tucked into a pocket and taken with you through your day, discreet and portable.

Steam Diffusion

Steam diffusion is another method. You can boil a few cups of water and pour it into a bowl. Several drops of the oil will be placed into the bowl. The fact that the water is already hot will keep the water releasing steam into the air. However, this steam will now carry the essential oils with it; this is a relaxing way to use aromatherapy and be a perfect complement to a spa treatment or a massage treatment.

Candle diffusion

In this method, you light a candle and allow it to burn for a few minutes. After a little while, put out the candle and place a drop of the oil into the melted wax and then relight the candle. Be very careful, as essential oils are highly flammable! You want to keep the oil in the wax and not near the flames to prevent them from catching on fire.

Reed diffusion

This is an increasingly popular method of diffusion. In this method, a reed is placed into a bowl of diluted essential oils. The reed soaks up the oil material, and the liquid runs upwards along the reed itself. As the liquid moves, it diffuses the oil particles into the air.

Fan diffusion

This can also be quite effective. In this method, a fan diffuser uses the fan to blow the essential oil into the air. The fan blows across a disposable pad or tray that is placed within the overall system. The air blown from the fan carries across the tray, lifting particles of the oil into the air.

Other methods

There are many other types of diffusers in the market. They vary in size, complexity, and in the strength of the aroma released into the 30

room. Some are more personal for you to carry on your person while others easily handle an entire room. Some will produce a greater concentration than others, and so it is best to review the different types of diffusers to make up your mind as to which one is best for your use.

CHAPTER 14

HOW SHOULD ESSENTIAL
OILS BE STORED?

One crucial key fact to note about essential oils is that they do not go wrong. Therefore, storing them can be pretty simple with some careful precautions. They are commonly sold in small bottles, but if you are making your blends, you can find different-sized bottles to use (keep in mind that if your mix has a perishable oil in it, this limits your ability to store it).

While essential oils do not go wrong, they can lose their effectiveness and deteriorate. Some oils may even oxidize and lose both aroma and therapeutic benefits, but this is not true for all lubricants. It is best to keep your oils in a translucent (but not transparent) bottle.

Amber or blue bottles are best for this because they will diffuse the light to try to get into the oils. Dark glass is always best for storing all of your aromatherapy items, particularly those, which can cause phototoxicity as they are more susceptible to the adverse effects of light.

It is such an issue that you use dark glass not to purchase oils sold in clear containers. You will not ascertain how long this oil was in a clear container, and it could have been exposed to light and lost its potency already. Look out for containers that use rubber stoppers as well. While this may seem highly convenient, a rubber stopper can get turned gummy from the highly concentrated oil and should always be kept out of the bottle itself. Keeping this oil in a bottle will ensure that you do not get access oil breakouts.

Another critical thing to be aware of is that aluminum bottles can be used for storing as long as they are linked on the interior. Anything that is not lined should not be used.

Keep your essential oils in the dark, fabulous location where they are away from the sunlight and kept at a relatively low temperature (not refrigerated or frozen). This is the best way to ensure they will last as long as possible. Heat is likely to accelerate deterioration, like sunlight, which can cause your oils to go wrong.

CONCLUSION

Aromatherapy has become a prevalent treatment method in the world of alternative medicine. It has become dominant and influential in areas where there are problems relating to emotions – such as stress and depression.

Within the detail of this book, I have told you about many of the different aromatic products available, and what to avoid, and the many other methods of applying these materials.

I hope that armed with this information, you will now enjoy the benefits that aromatherapy can bring to your life.

Good luck!

CPSIA information can be obtained
at www.ICGtesting.com
Printed in the USA
BVHW080943120521
607048BV00009B/2945

9 781802 867718